A JOURNEY OF HOPE AND DESPAIR :

A CARER'S EXPERIENCE AND PERSPECTIVES WITH PROSTATE PATIENT

Godfrey Hunt

Table of Contents

Chapter 1

The Early Days

This book is a personal account of the experience of caring for an old male who was diagnosed with benign prostatic hyperplasia (BPH), also known as a prostate disease when he was in his late 80s. For the sake of this narrative, we shall refer to him as Sir Barry. The account takes place between the diagnosis and the patient's last day on earth in the hospital during a 1-year, 8-month timeframe. The setting was Southeast Nigeria, with its peculiar poor healthcare care system, but the takeaways have global relevance and so I would urge you to read on, irrespective of your geographical peculiarities.

Sir Barry was my father, and my name is Godfrey. He had always managed his hospital appointments, making routine visits as at when due, as long as I could remember. When it became clear that he could no longer manage those hospital appointments on his own, I had the honor of being one of his caregivers who assumed responsibility for making sure the appointments were kept. You might find it interesting to know that Sir Barry had suffered from heart disease and high blood pressure for the past 30 years, making him a frequent outpatient during that time.

Before February 2013, Sir Barry would spend an excessive amount of time trying to empty his bladder and bowels when he went to the bathroom. I must admit that since I didn't live where he did, I couldn't tell you exactly when this problem started. He preferred living in the country, only visiting the city to pick up supplies or for doctor's appointments, or some other meetings.

Let me give you a brief introduction to Sir Barry. Back in his day, he was a charismatic community leader. He raised six surviving children who all contributed to his care.He didn't back down from a fight and would confront you to resolve the disagreement. He was a proud and modest man. So you can you imagine having to talk to anyone else about matters concerning his genitalia? That, I would suppose, led to the delay in informing his children of the escalating situation. How do you have a conversation about a man's genitalia with him when he is an adult and hasn't told you anything? The presence of Sir Barry caused such an aim to fail. When you sat down with him, you would prefer to talk about something else. He was that kind of a man. Or, were we carried away by his independence of mind, that we failed to engage thoroughly him on his healthy. We were used to seeing him go to hospital and come home with his drugs. His vibrancy even in his eighties somehow fulled us.

So it came as a surprise, when his wife Lady Barry, my mother, called me in the middle of February 2013 to ask me to take the elderly man to a urologist.

Sir Barry didn't think highly of the doctor that day at the urologist's office, and it's hard to blame him. Without appropriate

sensitization regarding how the probing will be done and what was the target, the doctor inserted two fingers in Sir Barry's anus. With any other person, you might get away, but not Sir Barry. He kicked the doctor in the thigh as the examination was going on. The doctor was a little frustrated, and I didn't want a situation where we had to deal with an angry doctor, so I had to settle things down. The doctor later implanted a urethral catheter to relieve the bladder's urine retention after the evaluation. Sir Barry felt less discomfort, yet he still had some mixed emotions. He had just started a road of humiliation thrust on him. While I was driving him home, he didn't say anything, but I understood his silence. Two drugs that are intended to reduce the size of the enlarged prostate were recommended by the doctor. After getting the medication, we left for home. A weekly catheter change was requested by the doctor.

A look at some information about the prostate before we wrap up this section, wIll be relevant for the purpose of this text .

One of the glands responsible for producing the fluid that delivers sperm during ejaculation is the prostate. The urethra, the tube via which urine exits the body, is encircled by the prostate gland.

The gland has expanded if the prostate is enlarged. Almost all men have prostate enlargement as they age.

BPH, or benign prostatic hyperplasia, is another name for an enlarged prostate.

It is unclear what causes prostate enlargement. The development of the gland and testosterone levels may be influenced by aging-related factors and changes in the testicular cells. BPH does not occur in men who had their testicles removed when they were young (for instance, due to testicular cancer).

Additionally, the prostate starts to get smaller if the testicles are taken out after a man develops BPH. This is not, however, a typical course of treatment for an enlarged prostate.

Let's examine some information regarding prostate enlargement:

With age, there is a higher chance of acquiring an enlarged prostate.

Because BPH is so widespread, it has been asserted that if men live long enough, they will all develop an enlarged prostate.

Many men over the age of 40 have slight prostate enlargement. In men over 80, the illness affects more than 90% of them.

Other than possessing healthy testicles, there are no known risk factors.

When the prostate gland's cells start to multiply, it happens. Your prostate gland swells as a result of the extra cells, pressing the urethra and decreasing urine flow.

BPH doesn't enhance your chance of cancer and is not the same as prostate cancer. But it can also result in symptoms that lower your quality of life.

BPH affects a lot of males over 50.

BPH is seen as a typical aging issue. Although the exact cause is uncertain, aging-related alterations in male sex hormones may play a role.

BPH symptoms are frequently relatively modest at first but if left untreated, they might worsen. Common signs and symptoms include

- incomplete bladder emptying
- the need to urinate two or more times each night
- nocturia, which is marked by dribbling at the end of your urinary stream
- incontinence, or urine leakage
- straining when urinating
- a weak urinary stream
- an urgent urge to urinate
- painful urination
- and blood in the urine

If you experience any of these symptoms, consult your doctor. They can be treated, and frequent treatment can help avoid problems.

Your doctor will often conduct a physical examination and inquire about your medical history before testing you for BPH. During the physical examination, the doctor will perform a rectal examination to determine the size and shape of your prostate. Other examinations might be:

- In urinalysis, both blood and bacteria are examined in your urine
- test for urodynamics
- PSA test, or prostate-specific antigen test (This blood test looks for prostate cancer)
- leftover after voiding (This gauges how much urine is still in your bladder after urinating)
- Cystoscopy (This involves using a tiny, illuminated scope that is placed into your urethra to examine your urethra and bladder)

Your physician might also inquire about any drugs you're taking that could be affecting your urinary system, such as:

- antidepressants

- diuretics
- antihistamines
- sedatives

Any medication changes that are required can be made by your doctor. Never try to change your medicine or dose on your own.

If you've tried self-care for your symptoms for at least two months and haven't seen any change, let your doctor know.

Self-care and alterations in lifestyle can be the first steps in BPH treatment. If symptoms don't go away, doctors might advise medication or surgery. The recommended course of treatment will also depend on your age and general health.

Back to Sir Barry, the doctor ordered a prostate-specific antigen (PSA) test and an ultrasound scan. The PSA test result returned a value of 4.5 ng/mL (nanogram per milliliter). The family's biggest concern at this time was the possibility of dealing with prostate cancer. Though the PSA result was slightly higher than the normal range, and there is a consensus that the higher the values the higher the chance of developing prostate cancer, again, it is not definitive. So the doctor advised that to be certain about what is happening to his prostate, a prostatic biopsy would need to be performed. I will tell you more about the decision later on.

Chapter 2

Urinary Tract Infection And Other Problems

Persistent urinary tract infections brought on by repeated catheter use and bladder retention were one of the main problems I had to deal with while providing care for Barry.

Let's talk about infections that affect the prostate using data from the literature.

When your prostate and the surrounding tissues become inflamed, you get a prostate infection (also known as prostatitis).

The prostate can be infected in many different ways. While some men with prostatitis report having no symptoms at all, others say they have several, including excruciating agony.

Prostatitis can be of four different types:

The rarest and shortest-lasting type of prostatitis is acute bacterial prostatitis. In addition, if untreated, it may be fatal. The diagnosis of this kind of prostatitis is the simplest.

The second is chronic bacterial prostatitis, which manifests gradually over many years with less severe symptoms. Recurrent urinary tract infections are more likely to occur in young and middle-aged males with this condition (UTIs).

The groin and pelvic region might also experience pain and discomfort due to chronic prostatitis or chronic pelvic pain syndrome, which is the third type. Men of any age can be impacted by it.

The fourth and final condition is known as asymptomatic inflammatory prostatitis. There are no symptoms despite the prostate being inflamed in this case. Typically, a clinician finds it while identifying another issue.

It's not always clear what causes prostate infections. The precise cause of chronic prostatitis is uncertain. According to researchers, a microbe can result in chronic prostatitis.

The cause of both acute and chronic bacterial prostatitis is bacterial infections.

Bacteria can occasionally enter the prostate through the urethra.

If you use a catheter or undergo the urethral procedure, your risk of developing a prostate infection is enhanced. Other danger signs consist of:

- sexually transmitted infections and bladder blockage (STDs)
- damage or an enlarged prostate, which can promote infection

Different types of prostate infections have different symptoms.

Acute bacterial prostatitis symptoms appear abruptly and are severe. Immediately seek medical help if you experience:

- stinging or discomfort while urinating
- the difficulty to empty your bladder
- body aches
- fever and chills
- abdominal or lower back pain

Additionally, you might smell something nasty or find blood in your urine or semen. or have excruciating lower abdominal pain or urination. These could be symptoms of a bacterial prostatitis infection that is acute.

A chronic infection's symptoms are less severe than an acute illness and may come and go. These symptoms either don't worsen or do so gradually and include:

- burning while peeing
- frequent or urgent urination
- pain in the groin
- lower abdomen or lower back pain
- bladder pain is a symptom that can linger for more than three months.
- pain in the penis or testicles
- difficulty initiating a urine stream or having a weak stream
- painful ejaculation
- UTI

The signs and symptoms of chronic bacterial prostatitis are similar to those of chronic prostatitis. Between your scrotum and anus, in the center of your lower belly, or the vicinity of your penis, scrotum or lower back during or after ejaculation are additional areas where you might feel uncomfortable or in pain for three months or longer.

If you experience painful ejaculation, painful urination, or pelvic pain, see a doctor.

Your medical history, a physical examination, and diagnostic testing are used to make the diagnosis of prostate infection. During the examination, your doctor can also rule out other severe illnesses, such as prostate cancer. Your doctor will perform a digital rectal exam while performing a physical examination to check for the following things:

- discharge
- huge or tender groin lymph nodes,
- swollen or tender scrotum.

Aside from your symptoms, recent UTIs, and the drugs or supplements you're taking, your doctor may also inquire about them.

Among the additional medical examinations that can aid in your diagnosis and course of therapy are

- urinalysis and semen analysis, which screen for infections
- a prostate biopsy or PSA blood test
- urodynamic testing to determine how your bladder and urethra hold pee,
- and cystoscopy to check for obstructions inside the urethra and bladder

To obtain a better look, your doctor can also request an ultrasound. The proper course of treatment will be determined by the cause.

Before using complementary or alternative medicine, always consult your doctor. Herbs and supplements may interact with prescription drugs you are already using.

If you are exhibiting signs of prostate infection, consult your doctor. These could include lower back or groin pain or discomfort when urinating. To begin treatment, it is preferable to receive a diagnosis as soon as possible.

And so with Sir Barry, urinalysis and sensitivity culture test conducted on his urine samples produced significant growth of Escherichia Coli, a gram-negative bacteria. I was made to understand by the doctor, that the indwelling catheter was a major predisposing factor for the infection. According to the Center for Disease Control and Prevention (CDC), about 75% of UTIs developed in a hospital are connected to a urinary catheter. For most of the time, clearing Sir Barry's infection was an uphill task. Strong antibiotics were frequently used. During the bouts, his urine contained sediments and was cloudy most of the time.

Chapter 3

The Deterioration Of Memory And Other Conditions

By the middle of 2014, I was also dealing with Sir Barry's deteriorating memory and considerably diminished communication skills. Before this, in January 2014, Sir Barry was treated for anemia and UTI complications in the emergency hospital. After a two-week hospital stay, it took the infusion of two pints of blood and a flood of intravenous antibiotics to bring him back to life. I couldn't recall Sir Barry ever sleeping in the hospital before this time, ever in my life.

Relating to memory problems, I must also admit that it was challenging to pinpoint the exact time of commencement because I observed that his conversation significantly decreased, even on days when he felt less discomfort. I mistook his silence for the lack of motivation that comes with illness.

I would purposely start a conversation on subjects he frequently had an opinion on, but he would typically only reply by nodding in agreement and grinning most of the time. That's all there is to it. To get Sir Barry to respond, you would have to repeat the cycle. According to trusted sources, several illnesses can impair memory in elderly people. It's crucial to have a timely diagnosis and suitable care.

Aging is generally associated with some degree of memory issues as well as a mild reduction in other thinking abilities. However, there is a distinction between memory loss brought on by Alzheimer's disease and other related conditions, as opposed to alterations in memory that are normal. And some memory issues are the result of diseases that can be treated.

Normal aging-related memory loss doesn't significantly interfere with your day-to-day activities. You might occasionally forget someone's name but remember it later in the day, for instance. Sometimes you might lose your spectacles. To remember appointments or tasks, you might need to prepare lists more frequently than in the past.

Your capacity to work, live independently, or maintain a social life is not significantly impacted by these changes in memory since they are typically manageable.

A group of symptoms, including memory, reasoning, judgment, language, and other thinking skills impairment, are together referred to as "dementia." In most cases, dementia develops gradually, gets worse with time, and affects a person's capacity for work, social connections, and romantic relationships.

One of the first or more obvious indicators of dementia is frequent memory loss that significantly interferes with daily life. Additional warning indicators could be:

asking the same queries time and time again

using common terms incorrectly when speaking

confusing words

lengthier completion times for routine tasks, such as following a recipe

Putting things where they shouldn't be, like a wallet in a kitchen drawer,

getting lost when driving or strolling at a well-known location

undergoing unexpected changes in behavior or emotions

Among the symptoms mentioned above, Sir Barry showed forgetfulness and a decline in his ability to make sound decisions. He was no longer mobile on his own, so I couldn't tell if he knew how to get home.

On what could be responsible for memory decline, evidence in literature does not appear to concur that dementia or memory loss is directly related to prostate disease. While a study by Duan et al. connected taking the popular prostate medication to memory issues, others thought the study was insufficient to reach that conclusion because some students have demonstrated that the medication has a limited capacity to cross the blood-brain barrier and that a drug with such a limited capacity cannot significantly affect the brain. Sir Barry was heavily dependent on this medicine. According to the literature, severe urinary tract infections may contribute to disorientation in the brain. I am inclined to believe that a person's ability to think is compromised when they are ill. So, I cannot conclude what caused the memory issues, but it was present at the height of the disease. He was a completely different man some months back when he could manage himself.

I would like to emphasize that the prostate problem was made worse by heart disease, impaired kidney function, and persistent UTI. His breathing was labored, and his feet continued to swell. The family believed that these underlying issues made it unsafe to conduct a biopsy of the prostatic enlargement.

Sir Barry was a bulky man weighing about 205 pounds with a height of 1.6 meters. I believe his weight alone predisposed him to heart disease and appeared to be impacting negatively his heart condition. Managing his weight through special diets and reduced portions were adopted to help him take some weight off his heart.

Aside from other vital indicators, those moments were made hopeful when I glanced at his legs in the morning and noticed that they were lean without the swollen appearance. But I would notice symptoms of water retention developing on the legs as the day wore on. Those filled me with despair for Sir Barry, who was 88 at the time. Every improvement in his eating, mood, or appearance sent me on a high-flying optimism that the drug might be decreasing the big prostate. For me, it was a daily voyage of hope and despair. But by evening, I would give up when I noticed signs of fluid accumulation in the legs, which told me that his long-standing hypertension and a weak heart were complicating his recovery. I also got the feeling that the liver and kidneys were having a hard time keeping up with the number of medications his system was dealing with...

It could now seem as though some of these evident indicators were not investigated further, or even worse, it could give the impression that Sir Barry was not well taken care of. False. Although Sir Barry was surrounded by family members who cared for him and wanted to see him get well, some treatment choices were not an option for him due to underlying medical conditions he had for a long time. This was in the opinion of the family. The family decided they wouldn't allow him to have a biopsy because of his cardiac problem. The information available in the literature lists hematuria, rectal bleeding, pain in the hypogastrium, perineum, or urethra, fever, nausea, vomiting, urinary retention, or other negative reactions as potential side effects of a prostate biopsy. We didn't want to try this on an 88-year-old man. Therefore, a good care regimen made sure he had a healthy diet, practiced good cleanliness, never lacked company, and never ran out of medications or supplies. Nevertheless, despite everything, I sometimes discovered Sir Barry seated in his preferred chair with his head bent. I'll try and explain why in the following chapter.

Chapter 4

The Catheter Humiliation And Alternative Solutions Failure

Embarrassment and humiliation are similar, but humiliation usually lasts longer and hurts more. An urge to run away or hide can occasionally be used to describe humiliation. It has a strong connection to shame.

Never in all my years of caring for Sir Barry was there ever a procedure that traumatized me more than when he needed to wear a new catheter. Trauma, not because the procedure made me feel uneasy, but rather because of how it affected him and the message that was hidden on his face. He voiced it a few times. The most embarrassing situations he ever encountered were each catheter change. Every time he had to change it, he wished he had died. Unfortunately, he had to go through this every week. No amount of motivation or prodding would convince him of the need for someone, male or female, to handle his penis like a piece of equipment to implant the catheter. Even though he loved his daughter-in-law dearly and she was typically the one changing the catheter, nothing changed. He would comply when she would calm him down during the change so the tube could be positioned, but he was one of the saddest men at the moment. He was broken, as far as I could tell. As I discovered after his passing, while researching the psychological effects of catheterization, Sir Barry was not the only one who felt that way.

One individual who had to use the catheter for over 3 years due to problems with the bladder stated that he wished he didn't have to urinate via a catheter. He continued "I regret any mistakes I may have made that may have resulted in bladder dysfunction and the requirement for a catheter. I also regret having experienced such severe anxiety and sadness over my four and a half years as a catheter user." He summarizes that Although it is rarely discussed, catheterization can occasionally hurt one's mental and emotional well-being. While some persons may experience sadness or anxiety associated with catheterization, others may adjust to catheterization with little difficulty. Again, Psychreg.org states that a wide range of problems, including concern, overthinking, feeling like a victim, and shame, beset someone who has a protracted catheter dependence. In catheterized cohorts chosen for research on the psychological impact of catheter use, depression has been noted to be common in some catheterized patients.

Other studies claimed that using a catheter had an impact on their sense of self. A female subject, for instance, believed that her catheter prevented her from having a romantic connection.

In retrospect, he described the urethral catheter as a "blooming irritation" that he detested having.

Those of us who were close to Sir Barry were also impacted by his condition of despair, and we would do anything to see him recover and stop using the catheter. People of all stripes visited us at that time to try to offer us various remedies, including herbal items. I declined, telling Lady Barry that dad had to keep taking his medication schedule. Lady Barry bought into one of the alternate options being pushed as soon as I left the state on a trip. You have to imagine how expensive the herbal remedy was. A week later, when I returned from my trip, there was a terrible smell waiting for me. What was what? Because his medicine had to be interrupted to try the alternative herbal remedy, the UTI had gotten worse. The pee had a hint of blood and pus in it. Lady Barry's sense of smell wasn't particularly keen, maybe due to age. She was in her 80s, so she didn't notice anything unusual. There was a putrid smell when you first walked into the room. That is how we ended ourselves back in the hospital to get the infection treated. You don't need to know how terrible Lady Barry felt about her choice. The herbal remedy was divided into two components: a plant-based brew to drink and an ointment to apply to the groin area. With the benefit of hindsight, I concluded that the man who offered the herbal remedy merely exploited the old woman's despair.

The doctors put in a lot of effort during this hospital stay to get rid of the UTI that had developed. I closely examined the urine bag's contents throughout the medication and was relieved when it began to get clearer, showing that the infection was fading. We stayed for a week before going back home.

Chapter 5

The Passing And Lessons Learned

Sir Barry's vital signs were not going well by December 2014. His breathing grew more labored, his feet—which had been slender in the morning—were more frequently inflated, and his blood pressure level had increased. His appetite also diminished. He stated that he would only visit the doctor in January due to Christmas. Looking back, I believe he was aware that he wouldn't be returning home if he went to the hospital at any time. It was the season when grandchildren visited their country home, so he wanted to spend more time with his family. He was making an effort to be more engaging during this time. You could see that when a child came to him to complain about something a sibling had done. Even though it was tough for him, he would smile at the child and invite him or her to go find the offender. To be present in case any guests arrived, he would remain in the living room for longer. We had a wonderful Christmas and holiday season.

When you were done taking care of him, he would always say "thank you," despite the obstacles he had to face. He would sincerely thank you whether you gave him his medication or helped him enter and exit the bedroom.

On January 2nd, 2015, I took him to the hospital to see the doctor, and as expected he was admitted. The doctor ordered a battery of tests. The results came back two days later. He was put on oxygen to help his breathing but most times the Pulse Oximeter placed in his finger displayed marginal readings. The doctor said his kidney had failed and so will need dialysis. He only had two sessions of dialysis because on January 15th, 2015, his Pulse Oximeter reading started dropping and it was only a matter of time before the inevitable happened. As I watched the display dwindling, it was a mixed feeling swirling within me. Somewhat happy that his pain will soon end and the humiliation he felt with a urethral catheter, again sad that my dad was dying. But of the two, having taken an active role in his care in these two years, I wanted him to go because he had wanted it.

At exactly 10:15 AM on the same day, Sir Barry violently jerked, gasping for breath even while the oxygen was on, and I watched the pulse and oxygen levels drop to zero. He breathed his last by 10:16 AM. An experience that has stayed with me to this day.

This brings us to lessons that I learned looking after him. Male catheterization, specifically, can be difficult, especially in patients with enlarged prostate glands or other potentially obstructive conditions in the urinary tract. So the use of different kinds of the catheter could ameliorate the situation, talking about self-catheterization and intermittent catheter use. But Sir Barry's physical condition and state of mind effectively made this option impossible. For a younger person, it will be ideal.

To assist older people to adjust to living with a catheter, healthcare professionals must be sensitive to their life situations and individual needs rather than focusing only on catheter performance and complications. Talking about memory issues, it is normal that everyone forgets things at times. Perhaps you misplace your keys or forget the name of a person you just met. But watch out for a consistent pattern, especially if the condition we are discussing is present. Maintenance of excellent hygiene in the handling of the catheter and the entrance to the urinary tract is of utmost importance.

If you have an indwelling catheter within your urethra, you are likely to develop a Catheter-associated urinary tract infection (CAUTI).

Numerous pathways exist for bacteria or fungus to enter your urinary tract and result in a CAUTI:

following implantation of your catheter, if your drainage bag isn't cleansed thoroughly, if you don't clean your catheter frequently enough, and if bacteria from excrement gets on you.

Hands must be washed with water and soap, and hospital gloves are worn before and during the insertion and removal of the catheter. Just as mentioned earlier in the text, the orifice of the penis, or vagina as the case may be, must be thoroughly washed with water and soap before receiving the catheter.

In delivering palliative care for prostate patients, psychosocial issues and their amelioration should be just as important as treatment because a more complex situation worse than the disease could develop, thereby making a patient's recovery difficult. The psychological and emotional well-being of the patient and those caring for him or her is important. It centers around communication and how to encourage patients to express themselves about the disease.

Communication is equally vital in catching when your or your loved one's prostate starts changing. We must have that conversation and get comfortable discussing prostate health. Sir Barry's makeup and disposition made it difficult for him to understand that discussions around genitalia should be "normal". Armed with information, it wouldn't have been out of place to strike up the conversation with him despite the barrier, knowing that it was a burning issue. We could have had the conversation 10 years earlier.

Prevention, they say, is better than cure, so what do we do so as not to have a situation where we are forced to wear a catheter due to an enlarged prostate? We must take our prostate health seriously. I must confess that the experience was also traumatic for me, as I have pondered from time to time whether I will suffer the same fate as my father. You know, the gene thing.

Some precautions that I am taking include minimal intake of alcohol if I must drink, and eating natural fruits and vegetables. Taking regular exercises at least 3 times a week, and watching the excess skin around my tummy has become an obsession for me in order not to gain so much weight. Most important is getting a yearly prostate check by a doctor as we advance in age. If you smoke, you have an increased risk of cancer including prostate cancer, so the earlier one takes steps to quit smoking, the better.